I'm Made of
Bananas

For kids and grown-ups who've
forgotten why we should eat healthy

I'm Made of Bananas
Hilla Starovisky
Illustrated by Jessica Melo

Original edition editor: Einat Kedem
Graphic design: Kobi Franco Design
Graphic execution: Shira Menahem, Tamir Pomerantz
English translation: Hilla Starovisky
Editor, English version: Amy Betz , Jenni Goodchild
Botanical advice: Dr. Yuval Sapir, Tel Aviv University Botanical
Garden
Nutrition specialist overview: Shoshanna Harrari

Many thanks to the wonderful and talented people who
worked with me to create this book, to my beloved Mum
and Dad, family, friends, and all the angels who helped me
on the way.

Please send comments to MadeOfBananas@gmail.com
Learn more at **www.MadeOfBananas.com**

Hilla Starovisky · **Illustrated by Jessica Melo**

I'm Made of
Bananas

For kids and grown-ups who've
forgotten why we should eat healthy

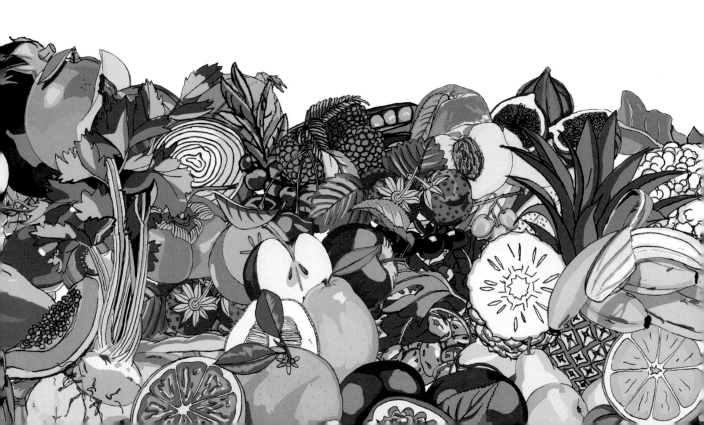

A Word to Parents

Studies have shown that most diseases, allergies and other conditions that are on the rise, such as cancer, diabetes, hyperactivity, depression, asthma, influenza, obesity, orthodontic problems, cavities, cataracts, hair loss, acne, inflammation, etc. can be completely avoided or improved by a diverse natural diet, especially with the consumption of raw food and green leafy vegetables. Many of these problems can be treated with natural remedies without running to the medicine cabinet, just as humans used to do for thousands of years.

The fascinating field of epigenetics (meaning "above the genes") reveals that with diet and lifestyle, we can make our less successful genes remain "turned off" and unexpressed, and thus gain mental and physical health and happiness.
While we are born with certain genes that are not under our control, it turns out that sometimes we are able to control their expressions. Like genes, epigenes are hereditary, so it is our responsibility to care for our children and grandchildren by maintaining a healthy lifestyle.

I always thought I was eating healthy, but the day I started eating a natural diet a "background noise" that had accompanied me for years stopped. From that day forward I have felt better in my body, and I have more strength and joy every day. I am thankful for this discovery and so I'm Made of Bananas was created to share this.

I'm Made of Bananas is suitable for anyone who wants to teach their children why it is important to eat healthily, and maybe even remember why themselves.

This book encourages us to take responsibility for what we put in our mouths, and explains some of the possible implications of our food choices. It may help with eating disorders. When the child understands the importance and meaning behind eating they become a partner in making better dietary decisions.

I'm Made of Bananas contains a lot of information. To be most effective, it is best to read this book in sections with your child. Each section is clearly marked, and there is also a bookmark.

The sections "Food Contains Nutrients" and "Listening to My Body" can be read while eating. The section "Preparing Food" can be read while preparing food, to increase the engagement of the child.

While reading a topic, make sure to discuss it with the child, to see how they experienced it; you may need to reread it until they understand. Perhaps you will even learn something new from their fresh perspective!

There is no mention of food sourced from animals because the issue is complex and inconclusive.

Reading **I'm Made of Bananas** may be appetizing... make sure you have some sliced fruits or vegetables prepared before you begin reading.
I'd love to hear from you at **MadeOfBananas@gmail.com**

Happy reading and enjoy!

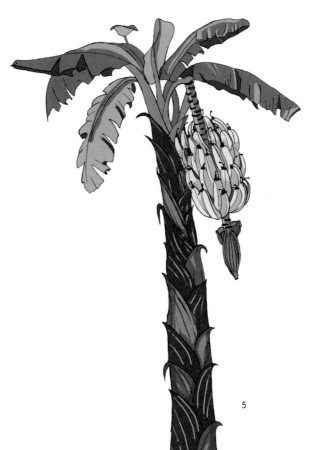

This book is about me and you and all
the children and grown-ups in the world.

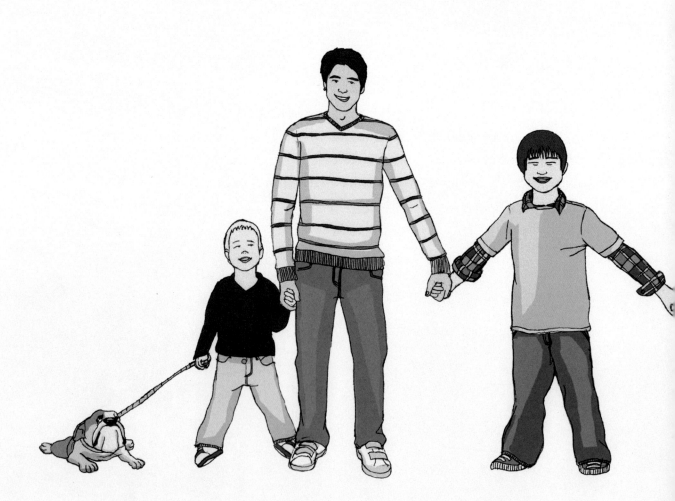

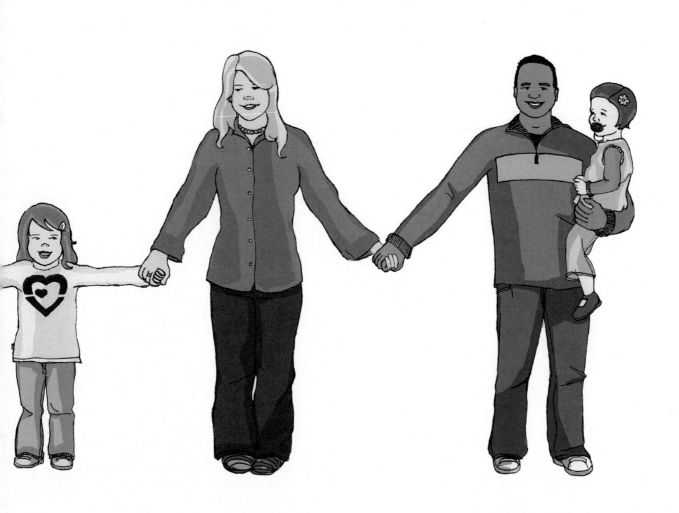

Everything is made of something.
Everything is built from something else.

What am I made of?
What builds me?
What materials build me?

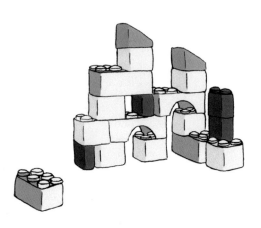

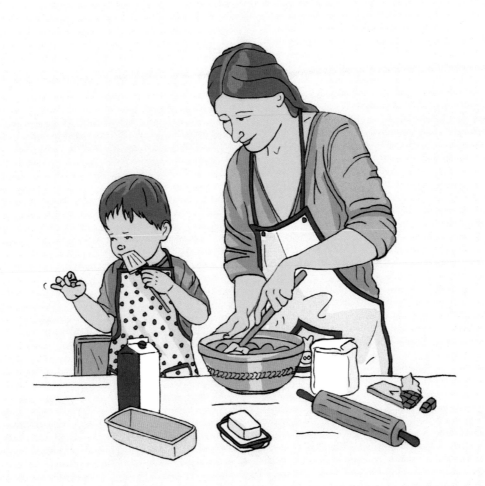

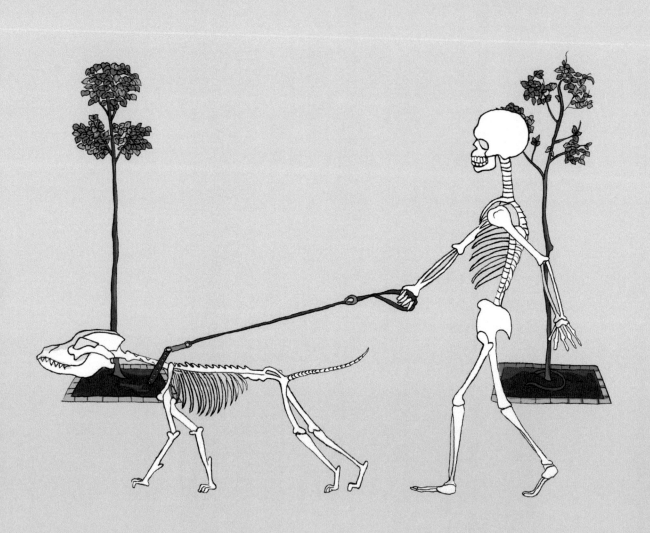

**Just like you, I too have a body.
My body is like a very clever machine
that does lots of things:**

It breathes.
It warms me up.
When I feel hot, it cools me down with sweat.
My body builds a lot of things for me:
It builds my skin,
My blood,
My bones,
My eyes,
My hair,
My nails,
My heart,
My stomach,
And my brain.
Everything in my body was built by my body itself,
without me telling it to.

My body renews itself constantly throughout my life. All the time, it is building things and breaking them down, building, and breaking down.

I am always brand new and fresh!

My hair grows long because my body builds new hair.

When I get a suntan, after a while my tan disappears because my body builds new skin and breaks down the old skin.

When I have a wound, my skin heals and the cut disappears because my body builds me new skin.

My nails grow long because my body builds new nails, and so sometimes I have to trim them.

My face changes. I become taller. My arms and legs become longer. Suddenly my clothes and shoes don't fit me anymore; they are too small and I need new ones. Without me noticing, just like magic, I am suddenly much bigger. I grow up and I change.

Even inside my body, the parts that I cannot see are being built, and broken down, and built, and broken down.

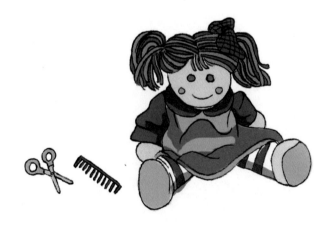

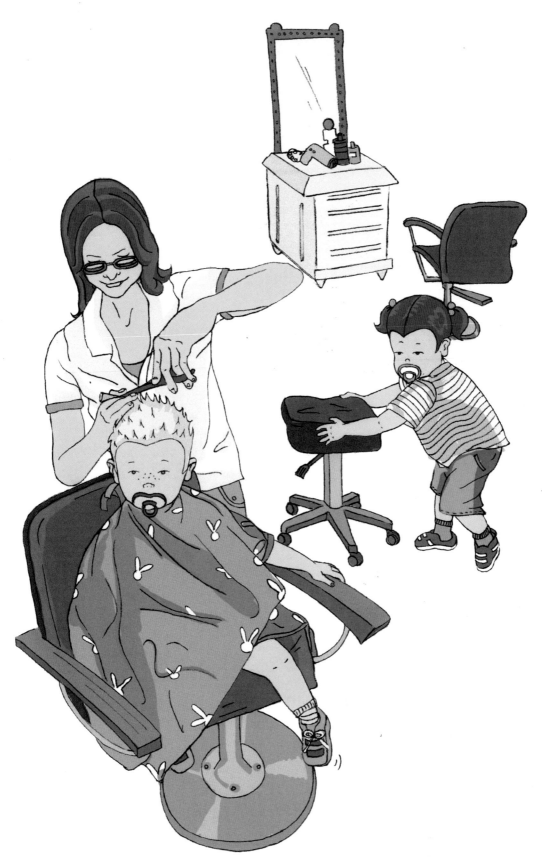

13

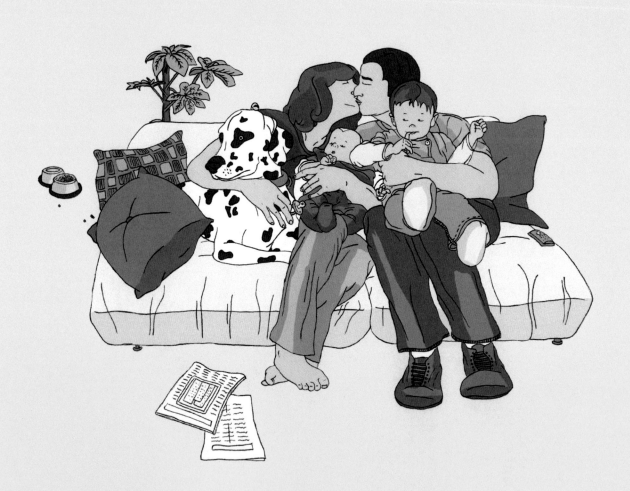

How do I help my body do these things?

I drink clean water.
I eat different types of food.
I breathe fresh air.
I go out in the sun for a short while.
I sleep and I dream.
And I give and receive lots of hugs and kisses
from loved ones.
By doing these things I help my body:
I drink, eat, breathe, go out in the sun, sleep,
and give and receive hugs and kisses.

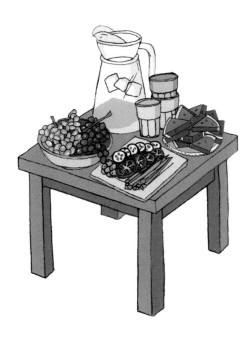

How do I help my body get rid of the stuff it has broken down and now no longer needs?

I go for a pee.

I go for a poop.

I blow out air when I breathe out.

I sweat.

When I have a cold and a runny nose, I blow my nose.

This is how my body disposes of the things it no longer needs.

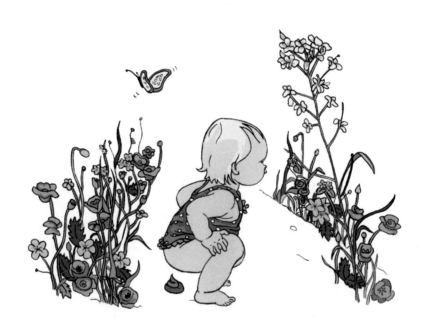

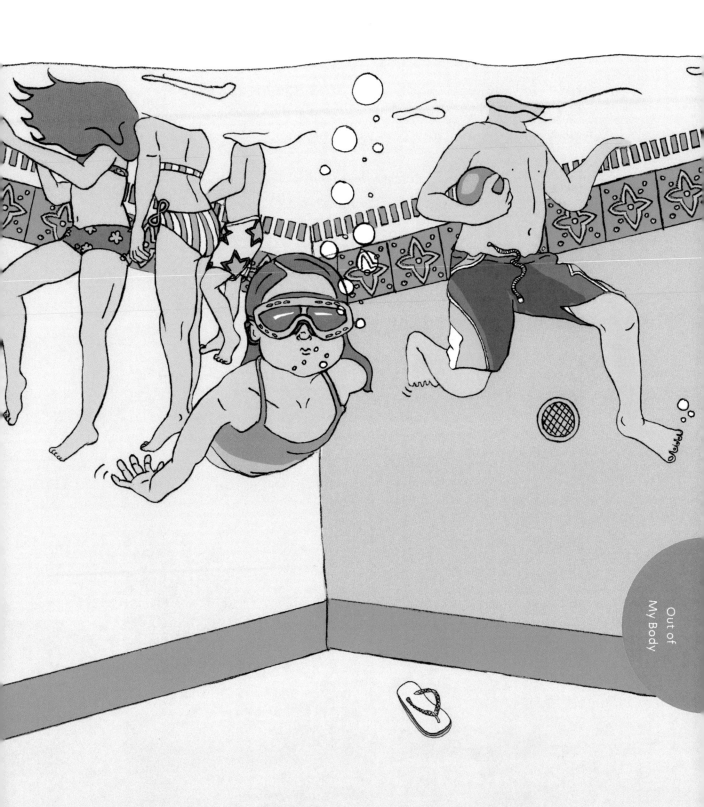

Nature has all the things that my body needs: sun, air, water and food.

Everything already exists and it's ready to use. There is no need to buy anything—simply reach out your hand and take what you need. It is all free and there is plenty for everyone.

There is plenty of sun and air. Water falls from the sky and flows in streams. Food grows on trees and on bushes.
In nature there are lots of plants. Some of them are poisonous and dangerous for us to eat, but are safe for other animals. Some of them are our food.

What kinds of food come from nature?

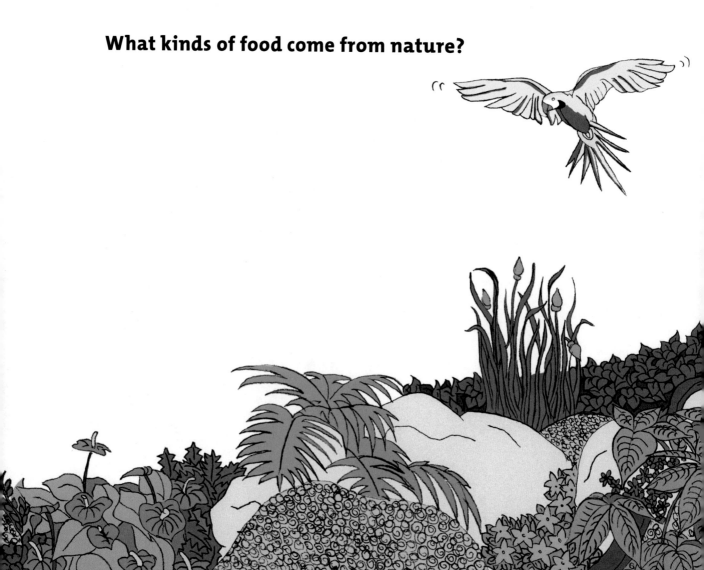

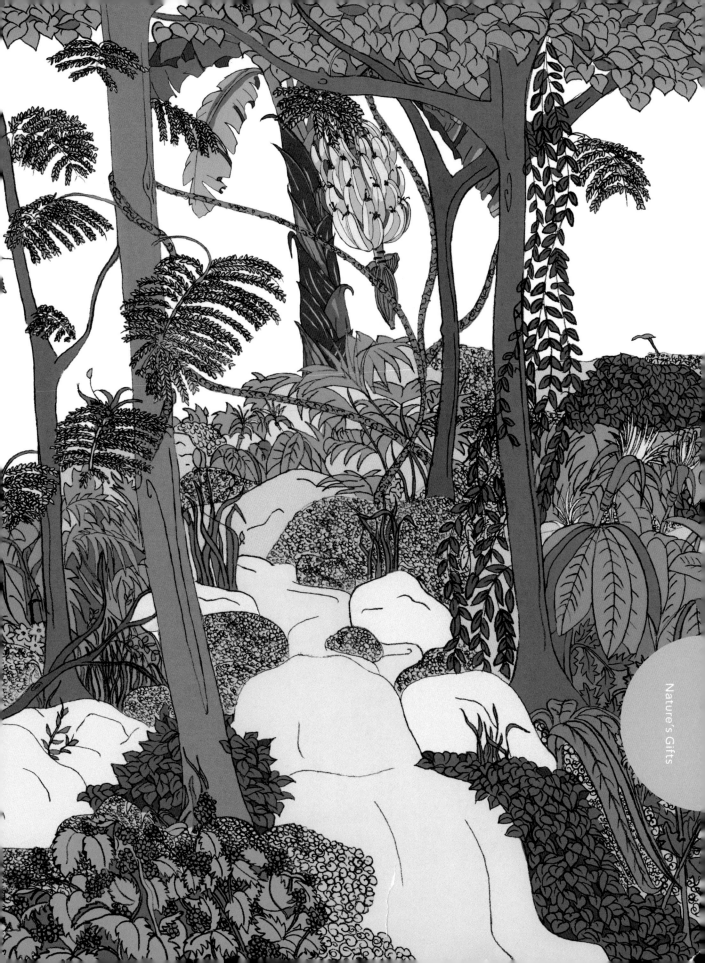

Nature's Gifts

Fruits

Fruits are the parts of a plant that contain seeds.
They taste sweet or sour and are rich in sugar.

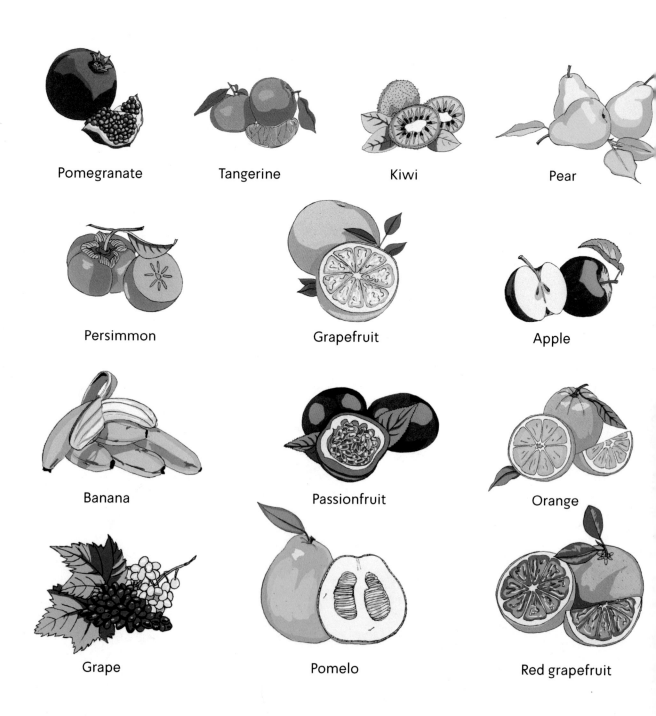

Pomegranate

Tangerine

Kiwi

Pear

Persimmon

Grapefruit

Apple

Banana

Passionfruit

Orange

Grape

Pomelo

Red grapefruit

What do you think tastes good?
What Fruits have you eaten today?

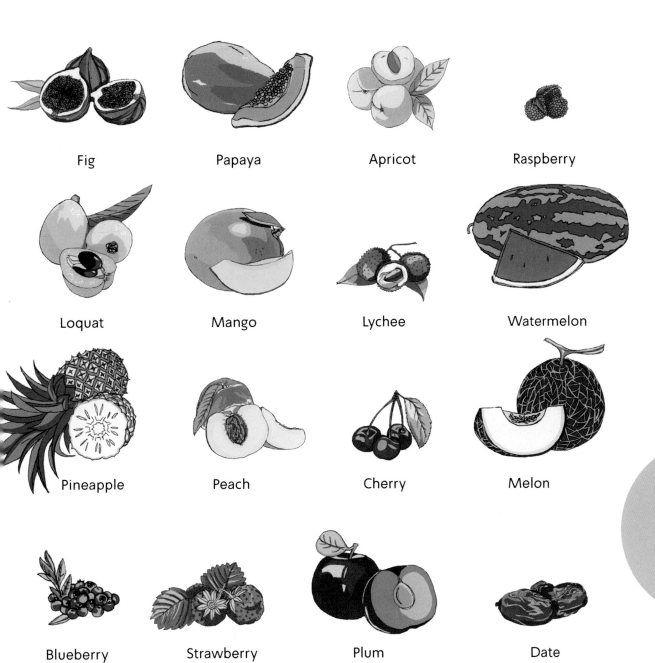

Fig

Papaya

Apricot

Raspberry

Loquat

Mango

Lychee

Watermelon

Pineapple

Peach

Cherry

Melon

Blueberry

Strawberry

Plum

Date

Vegetables

Vegetables are the edible parts of a plant and mushrooms.
Which do you like eating most?

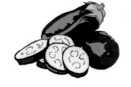 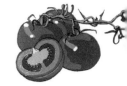

Fruits Eggplant   Tomato

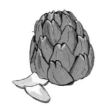 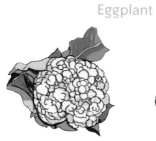 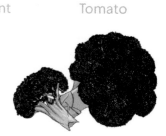

Flowers Artichoke   Cauliflower   Broccoli

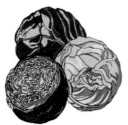 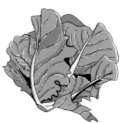 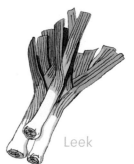

Leaves Cabbage   Lettuce   Leek

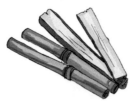 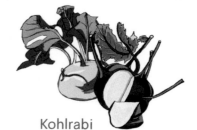

Stalks Sugarcane   Kohlrabi

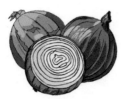 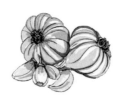 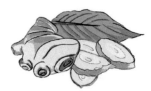

Roots / Tubers / Bulbs Onion   Garlic   Ginger

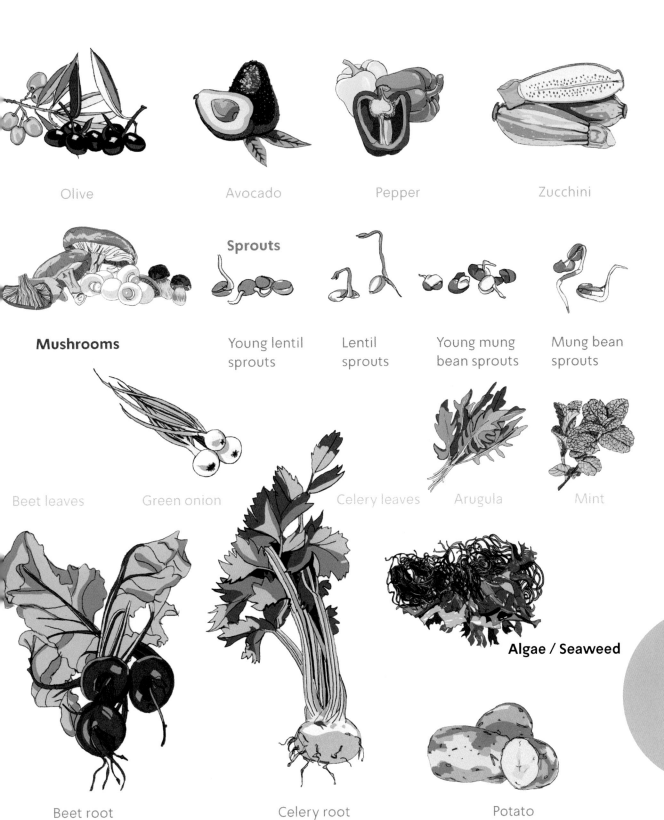

Olive

Avocado

Pepper

Zucchini

Sprouts

Mushrooms

Young lentil
sprouts

Lentil
sprouts

Young mung
bean sprouts

Mung bean
sprouts

Beet leaves

Green onion

Celery leaves

Arugula

Mint

Algae / Seaweed

Beet root

Celery root

Potato

Legumes

Legumes, also called pulses, have seeds that grow in a pod. They are rich in protein and can be used to make all sorts of things like spreads, burgers, noodles, stews, soups and salads. Or you can sprout them and eat them fresh.

What food do you know that has pulses in it?

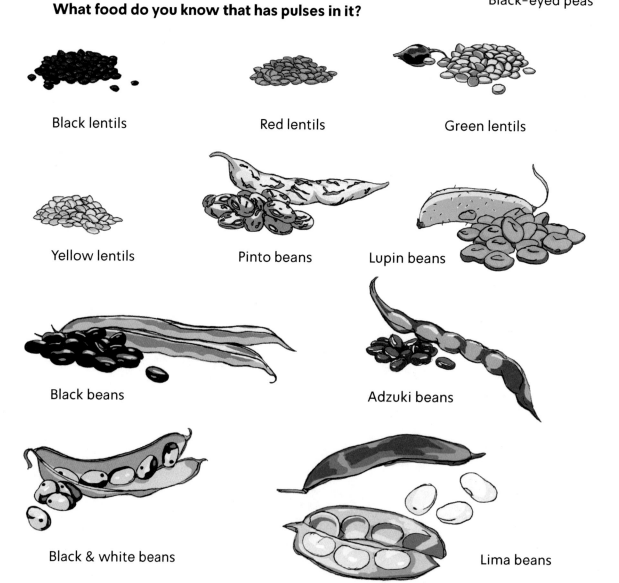

Black-eyed peas

Black lentils

Red lentils

Green lentils

Yellow lentils

Pinto beans

Lupin beans

Black beans

Adzuki beans

Black & white beans

Lima beans

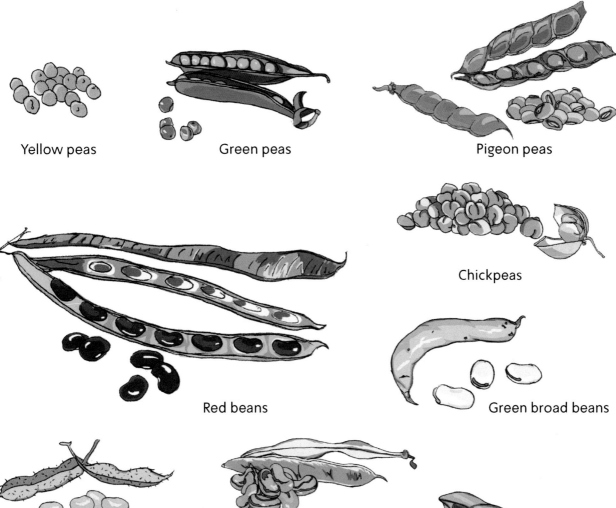

Yellow peas

Green peas

Pigeon peas

Chickpeas

Red beans

Green broad beans

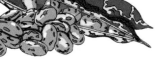

Soybeans

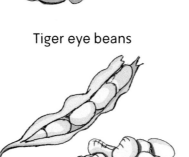

Tiger eye beans

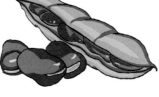

Red broad beans

Speckled beans

White beans

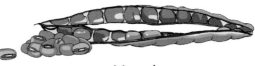

Mung beans

Grains

Grains are seeds that grow mostly in ears on stalks and are rich in carbohydrates. They are used to make flour for bread and pastries, noodles, pies, porridge, burgers, beer, liquor, milk, cheese, snacks, salads and cooked dishes.
Which haven't you tasted yet?

Cereal grain crops

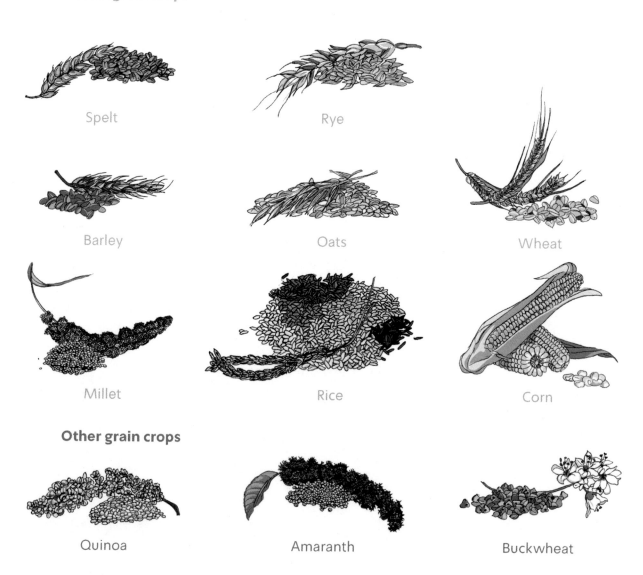

Spelt

Rye

Barley

Oats

Wheat

Millet

Rice

Corn

Other grain crops

Quinoa

Amaranth

Buckwheat

Nuts and Seeds

Nuts and seeds are seeds that usually grow in a hard shell and are rich in fats. They are used to make oils, spreads, candy, snacks, milk, ice cream and cheese.

What do you feel like eating right now?

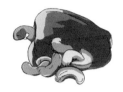

Cashew nuts

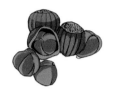

Hazelnuts

Flax seeds

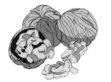

Walnuts

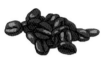

Coffee beans

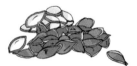

Pumpkin seeds

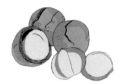

Macadamia nuts

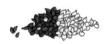

Sesame seeds

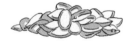

Watermelon seeds

Pine nuts

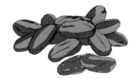

Cocoa beans

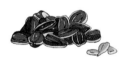

Sunflower seeds

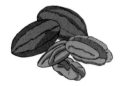

Pecans

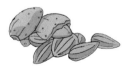

Almonds

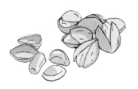

Pistachio nuts

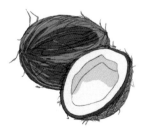

Coconut

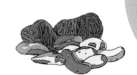

Brazil nuts

Nature's Gifts

My body needs lots of different materials to build me, to make me feel happy and to keep me healthy and protect me from being sick.

Everything I eat supplies my body with something. Any food that comes from nature contains things my body needs.

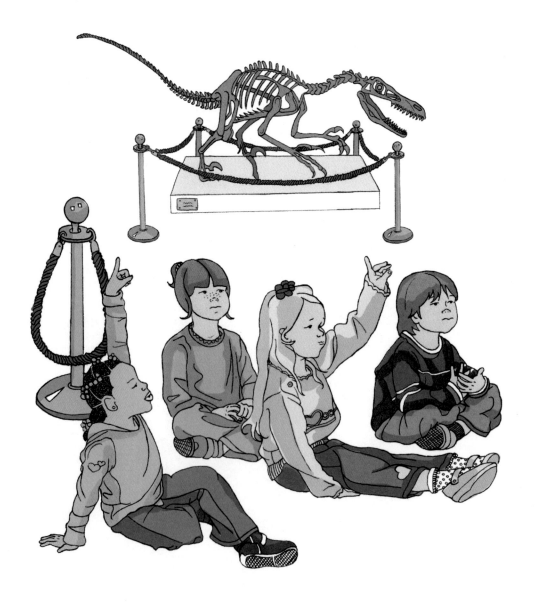

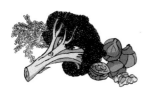

In seaweeds, walnuts, **dark green** leaves and vegetables like **Brussels sprouts, spinach** and **broccoli**, there is something called **omega-3** (which is a fatty acid). My body needs omega-3 for my brain and for keeping me smart and happy. If there isn't enough of it in my body, I might not remember things easily, or find it hard to learn new things. Without enough omega-3, I might not be patient or be able to pay attention for very long, and I might think more slowly or be sad for no reason.

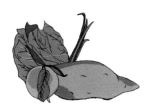

Vegetables that are yellow or orange or **dark green** contain something called **vitamin A** (which is a vitamin). My body needs it for my eyes, hair, nails and skin. If my body lacks this vitamin, I might not see very well and my skin might be dry and a bit stiff or I may have dandruff.

Vitamin A can be found in carrots, yams, peaches, apricots, pumpkins, **seaweed**, **spinach**, **green onions**, **parsley** and more.

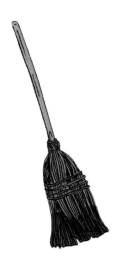

All leaves, whole grains, beans, vegetables and fruits contain **dietary fibers** (which are carbohydrates).

When they pass through my digestive system, they clean it, just like a broom or a scrub brush. Dietary fibers keep my digestive tract clear of materials that can cause diseases. They also help me feel full when eating and make my poop excellent: puffed, unified and soft.

Pulses, avocados, bananas and potatoes contain something called **potassium** (which is a mineral). My body needs potassium to make my muscles strong. If I lack potassium, I will feel weak and my muscles won't work very well.

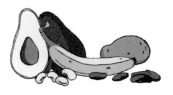

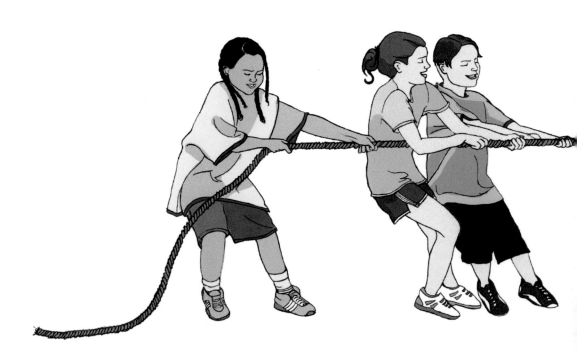

Natural foods contain the things my body needs: vitamins, minerals, enzymes, good bacteria (probiotics), food for the good bacteria (prebiotics), phytochemicals, antioxidants, dietary fiber, proteins, fats and carbohydrates.

Dark green leaves and vegetables contain something called **iron** (which is a mineral).

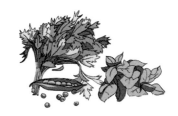

Iron can be found in **spinach, green beans, parsley, beet leaves, chard, grape leaves, dill, chives, basil, broccoli, seaweed, peas, asparagus, broad beans, soy** and more.

My body needs iron to grow and to give me power. If I lack iron I may be weak and get tired easily.

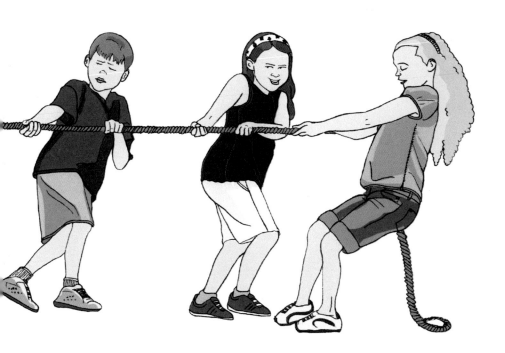

On top of **potassium**, **iron**, **vitamin A**, **omega-3** and **fiber**, my food contains many more important materials that my body needs. Some of them we haven't even discovered yet!

When the food I eat is fresh and I get it straight from nature, it has materials my body knows and needs.

Sometimes, a long time passes between the moment the food is good to eat and the moment I eat it. During this time, some of the good materials in the food disappear. This can happen if a nut I am eating was peeled a while ago, or a tomato I'm eating was picked a long time ago.

Sometimes, when preparing the food to eat, we do all sorts of things to it, like heat it. This can ruin some of the things in the food that my body needs.

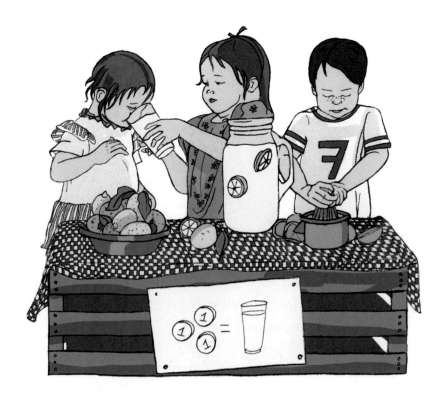

What sorts of things are done to the food when preparing it?

It is **chopped**,
when chopping vegetables to make a salad.

It is **squeezed**,
when squeezing oranges for juice or olives for olive oil.

It is **ground**,
when grinding wheat for flour or grinding sesame for tahini.

It is **fermented**,
when fermenting cucumbers for pickles, or when turning grapes into wine.

It is **steamed**,
when making steamed vegetables.

It is **cooked**,
when cooking a soup or a stew.

It is **roasted**,
when roasting vegetables on a grill.

It is **stir-fried**,
when stir-frying vegetables with noodles.

It is **baked**,
when making baked potatoes.

It is **fried**,
when frying French fries.

It is **radiated** with micro-waves,
when warming something frozen in the microwave oven.

It is **broken down** and important materials for my body are taken out, when making sugar from sugar cane, or making white rice out of natural rice, or making white flour from wheat or corn syrup from corn, or making potato starch from potato.

What food do you know that needs preparing?
Which of these actions do you think ruins more
things in the food and which ruins less?

Sometimes, when food is prepared, things that my body doesn't need are added.

Some of these things disturb my body. Then my body must work hard to clean itself, and we cannot always tell if it succeeds.

When something disturbs my body it can cause illnesses and symptoms like a headache, a runny nose, a rash, or tiredness. It can even make it hard to concentrate, create wounds, or make it hard to poop. Sometimes you notice it right away, or after a week, and sometimes only after years, when the damage has built up.

I try to make sure that nothing I eat will disturb my body. This way I help prevent diseases and unpleasant symptoms.

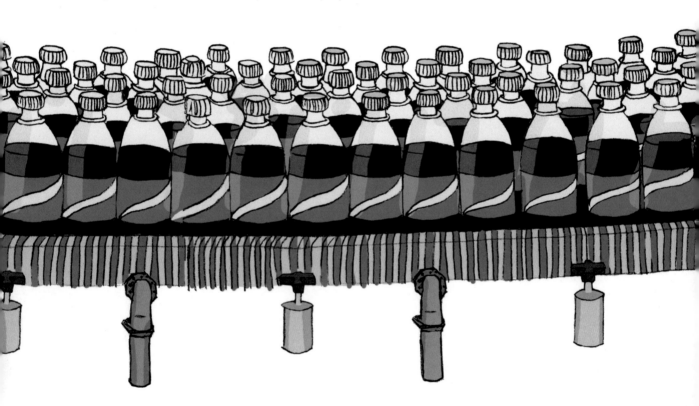

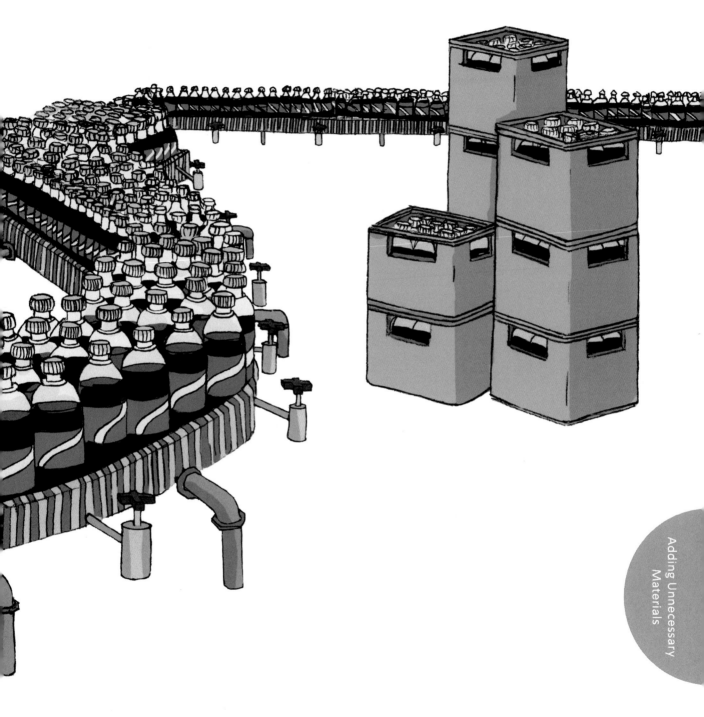

Why are things that disturb my body being added to my food?

To make food colourful and pretty, **food colouring** is added
like in popsicles, candy and coloured drinks.

To make food have a strong flavour and make us want more and more, **flavour enhancers** are added
like in salty snacks that are hard to stop munching.

To make food smell good and draw us to it, **fragrance** is added
like in grape juice made without grapes, or in popsicles.

To make food have an interesting shape, **stabilizers and gelatins** are added
like in jelly beans, marshmallows or ice cream.

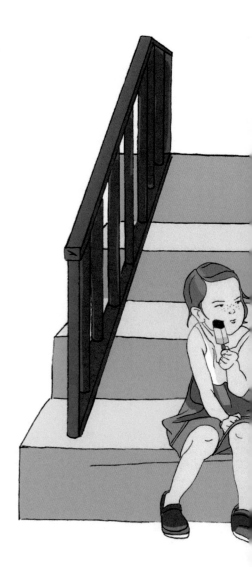

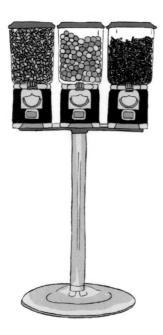

To make food edible a long time after it is made, **preservatives** are added
like in premade boxed spreads, salads or bread.

To make food sweet without adding sugar to it, **artificial sweeteners** are added
like sugar-free candy or yogurt.

To make food cheaper and last longer, **hydrogenated fats** or **trans fats**, are added, instead of butter or olive oil
like in cookies made with margarine.

Do you think these are good reasons for adding these materials?

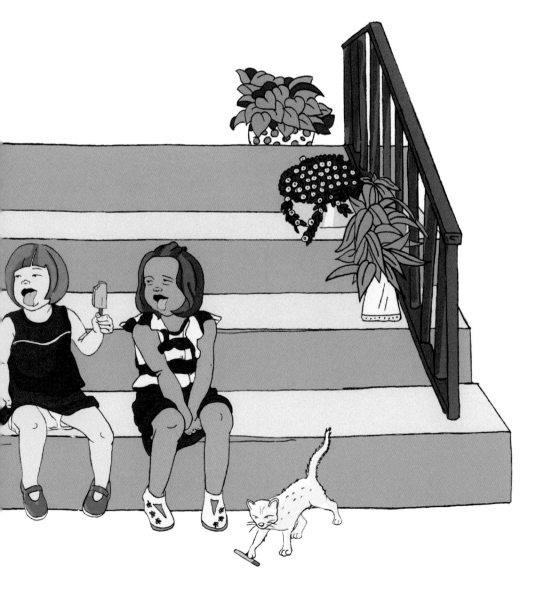

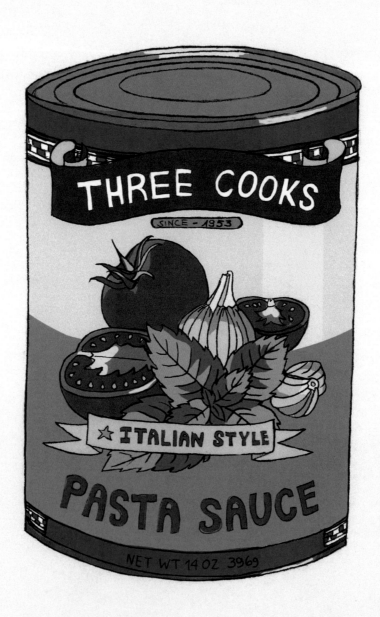

I like to read what is written on the packaging of the food I eat, because it lists the ingredients that went into making it.

The first ingredient is the one used the most in the food inside the package; the last is the one used the least.

On the list I see materials I know from nature like tomatoes, olives, and rice. These materials are good and natural for my body.

I might see materials I know from nature but they are not whole anymore because something was done to them — like sugar, palm **oil** or corn **syrup**.
There are also materials that were made in a lab. They do not grow on any tree or bush and I don't even know them from the supermarket.

These sorts of materials disturb my body and cover up the real taste of the food and make it hard for me to listen to my body.
Which ready-to-eat foods do you know that have added ingredients?

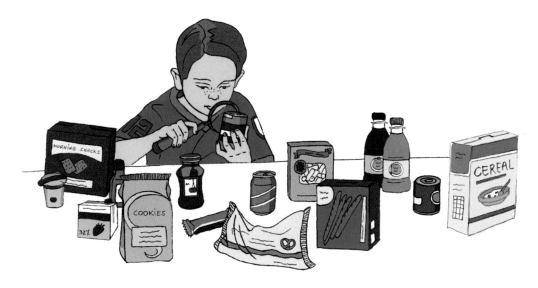

You may want to take a package of something and examine its list of ingredients together.
What is used the most? Which ingredients are not natural? Is it good for us?

Sometimes, food is also a medicine.

Once, when I got a small burn, we treated it by spreading honey on it, and it healed quickly.

When I had a cold, I ate lots of fresh peppers, kiwis and oranges, and the cold went away. Peppers, kiwis and oranges have vitamin C, which helps my body. Vitamin C is also the cure for a disease called the sailor's disease or scurvy. Scurvy happens when you don't eat food with vitamin C for a very long time.

Another time when I had a sore throat, it was inflamed, so we added some garlic to my salad, and soon the inflammation disappeared.
When I had sore ears, we dripped some warm olive oil in them, and the pain went away.

A medicine which is also food is sometimes called "folk medicine".
Since forever and until not too long ago, all the medicines that the doctor would prescribe were food or non-toxic plants that you could find in nature. It worked wonderfully in most cases. Even today, in most places in the world, food and plants are still used as medicine.

If I'm in pain or feel ill, the first thing I do is ask my mom if we can find a folk medicine online, and we look for it together.
Sometimes we ask folks around us; they seem to know some folk medicines without looking anywhere.

What folk medicines do you know?

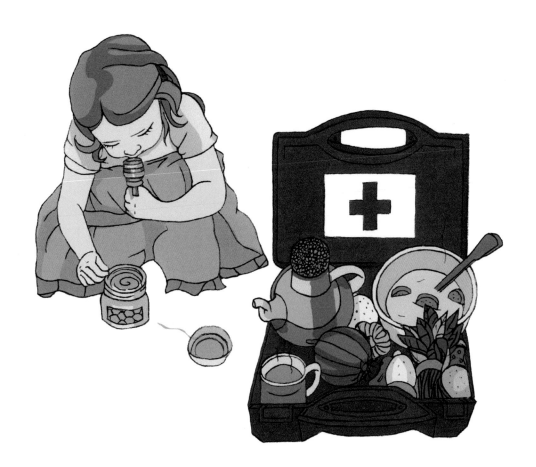

When I am healthy and my body has everything it needs, I look good!

My hair is full and shiny, my skin is fresh and smooth, my nails are strong and pretty, I smell good and I feel good being in my body. And then people even tell me, "Wow, you look good!"

When I am ill or when my body is missing something, I don't look very good, and people might say, "Oh dear, you look ill..."
You can tell from the outside what is going on inside my body.
The healthier I am, the better I feel and the better I look!

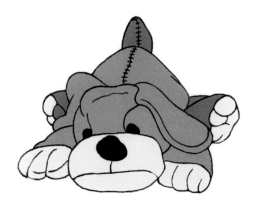

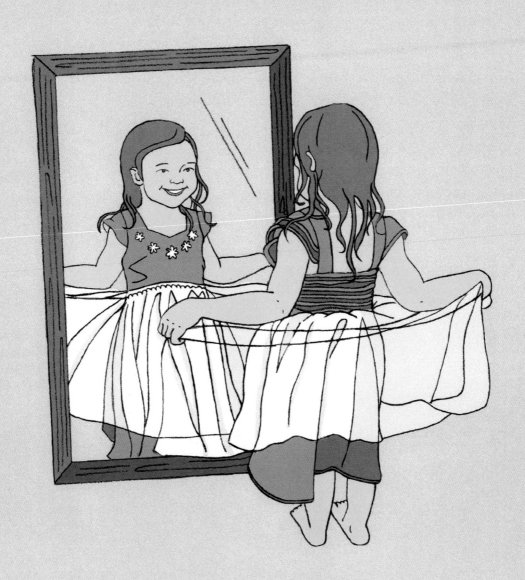

I eat all sorts of foods so that my body gets vegetables AND fruits AND grains AND pulses AND nuts and seeds.

I vary my food. This way my body gets everything it needs.

Sometimes my body needs something, and gives me clues to what it needs.
I just look at the food and already I know what my body needs.
I really know what I do and what I don't feel like eating.
Sometimes I want a tomato rather than a carrot.
Sometimes I prefer a carrot over a tomato.
And sometimes I just feel like eating a cucumber.
I take the cucumber in my hand and I can feel
if it is hard or soft, bumpy or smooth.

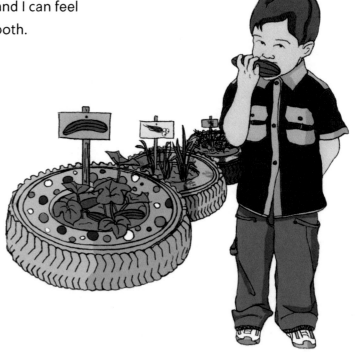

This part is best read while holding and eating
vegetables or fruits: lettuce, a sliced carrot,
pepper, apple, watermelon, orange,
some grapes etc.

When the cucumber is ready, and wants me to eat it, it lets me know by spreading an attractive scent.

I bring it close to my nose, smell it and check if I like the smell. I look at it.

If it looks yummy, I bring it to my mouth and bite it. And then I hear it crushing in my mouth and feel its taste with my tongue. The saliva in my mouth helps to break down the cucumber, and so do I.

I chew it well — chew, chew and chew — until the chewed cucumber becomes like a soup in my mouth, and then I swallow it.

My body finds it easy to take food apart only if I chewed it very well.

If the first bite was tasty, I take another bite. I eat slowly, take my time and enjoy the cucumber.

When I've had enough to eat and my body has enough food, I can feel it. I am no longer hungry, I feel content and I don't need to eat anymore.

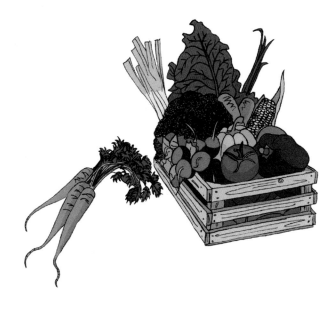

Sometimes it is hard for me to stop eating, even though I'm no longer hungry.
The food is so tasty and I want to keep enjoying it, and I feel that I can eat more—
until I am totally full.
But this is not a good idea, because after a little while I don't feel very good. I feel tired. This
is because eating too much is not good for my body; it disturbs it.
As if my body is saying to me, "We had too much to eat. Now there is a problem."
Just like if I take a huge bite, with a full mouth, I almost cannot chew; the same
happens in my stomach, which looks like a sack. If it is too full, it finds it hard to break down
the food inside.

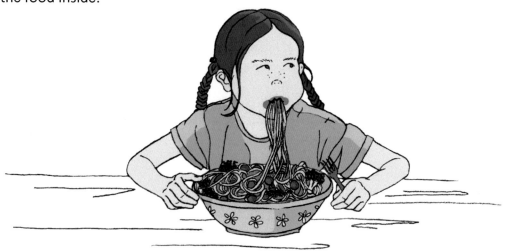

It is hard on the body to break down a lot of food at the same time. And when
something is hard on the body, it can cause diseases and symptoms.
This is why I always try to stop eating when I feel I am not hungry anymore,
even when the food is really tasty.
I have a trick. When I am no longer hungry, I say, "That was very tasty, thank you!" and I
push the plate far away from me, or I go and play. This way I keep feeling good. After
a few seconds, I even forget that I wanted to eat more.
Sometimes, this is hard for me to do, but most of the time it is easy and I succeed.
I know that if I am hungry again later, I can always eat more.

Sometimes I am excited about something so I cannot eat a thing. My hunger just disappears. Other times I eat without even being hungry.

- I eat because I'm bored and the food entertains me for a bit, but afterward, I'm bored again.
- Sometimes I eat because I'm sad, and the food comforts me for a while and it feels nice.
- I eat when I'm nervous and unsettled; the chewing calms me down a bit.
- I eat to get cooler or warmer, like eating a cold melon on a hot day or a hot soup on a cold day.
- Sometimes I'll eat because I'm thirsty, and will choose foods that contain a lot of water, like some watermelon or an orange.
- Sometimes I'll eat something because it is there in front of me, or because I've seen it a lot on commercials.
- At times I eat something in a particular time, out of habit, like eating dessert, even though I don't always really feel like it.
- Sometimes I eat because I am tired.
- At times I'll eat when what I really need is a hug.

I try to notice why I am eating when I eat. If it's not out of hunger, I'll see if there is something else I can do that would help me better instead of eating. For instance, I close my eyes, breathe deeply and relax, or go for a walk outside, have a nap, watch a funny film, dance, sing a song I love, or meet up with friends.
Or... I just eat and enjoy every bite!

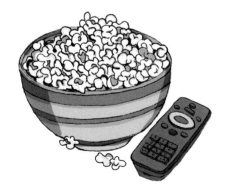

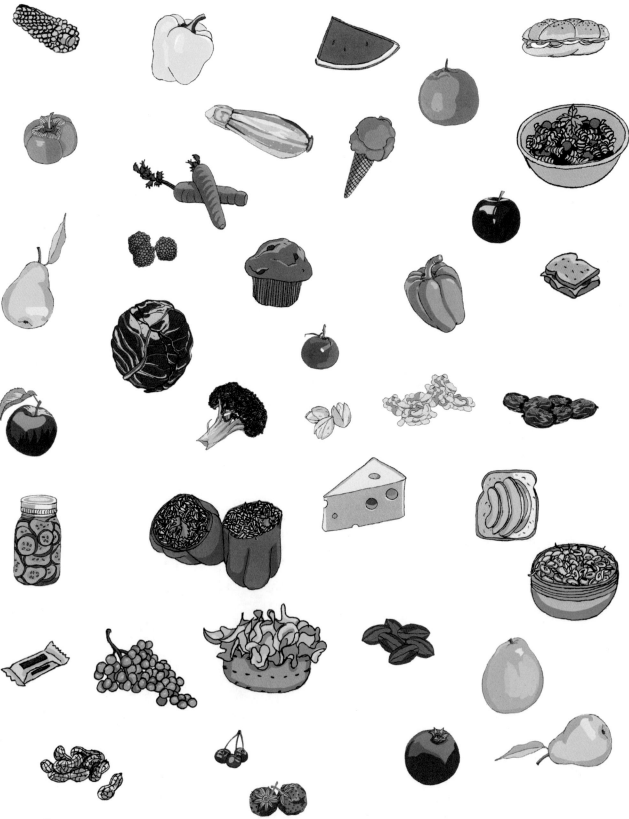

When I am very hungry, I feel like eating everything!

It feels as if my body is saying, "Bring me food! Now!"
Every food I see, I want, and everything looks delicious.

If I am very hungry and I am at a food shop, I feel like eating anything that is
ready to eat right now: chocolate, ice cream, candy, or salty snacks.
If I am very hungry and I am at a restaurant, I feel like ordering everything on
the menu: pizza, pasta, and steamed vegetables.
And if I am at home, I feel like eating everything that is ready to eat:
dates, strawberries, vegetable quinoa, lentils, or broccoli.

But then I am told, "Hey! Slow down. You're eating with your eyes. Your eyes
are bigger than your stomach."
This means that I cannot really eat all this food.
My eyes are big and want everything, but my stomach is small
and can only contain some of the food.

So first I eat what I am told is "real" food and is filling, like
lentils, vegetables or pasta, and only after I've finished
eating that, if I am still a little hungry, I eat a snack or
dessert like strawberries or dates.
To avoid getting too hungry, I eat a snack
every few hours: an apple, some carrots,
bean sprouts or a rice cake with a spread.

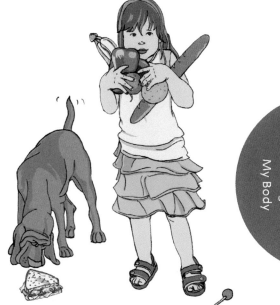

Every food that comes from nature, like an orange, is a perfect beautiful bundle of good materials that my body needs.

When I give my body natural foods, it is easy for me to feel when I have eaten enough and my body doesn't need any more food.

Fruits for example, are a natural food. I can only eat some—an orange, an apple, some grapes—and I feel full, because the amount and type of materials that are in the food are just right for my body.

Chocolate, however, is not a natural food. It is man-made. Chocolate is made up mainly of fat and sugar, and so it is best to have just a little. But I can easily eat loads of it without feeling fed up or being full, even though that is not good for my body. My body doesn't need loads of chocolate.

It is best for me to eat natural foods. If I eat mostly natural foods I will not get too fat or have cavities in my teeth.

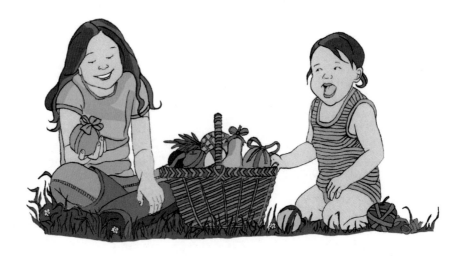

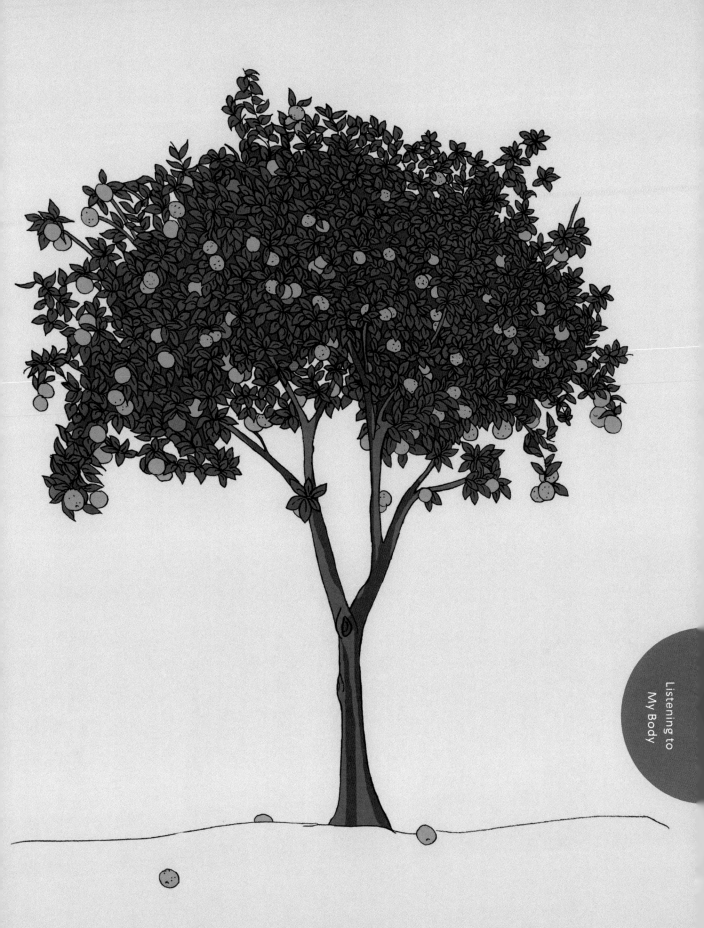

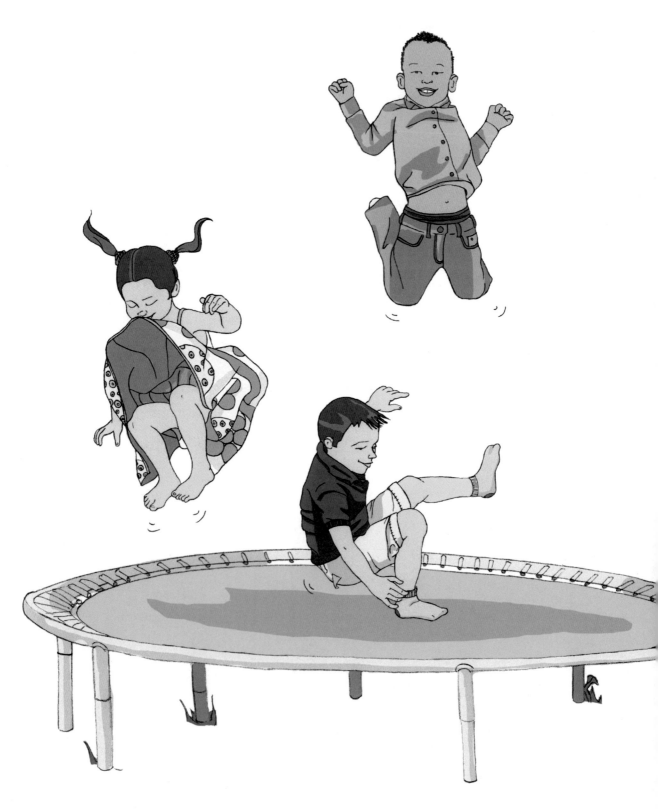

I love myself.

And I protect and care for me and my body.

The fruits and vegetables I eat protect me.

I ask, "What am I eating? Where did my food come from?

What was done to it after it grew in nature?"

I eat the freshest and most natural food, so that I will be made of the best materials.

I'm made of bananas, and rice, and peas and all the things I love to eat.

What are you made of?

I ask myself if I have had fruits and vegetables of the color orange this week.

And red? And green? And purple? And white?

When I give my body everything it needs, I have the power and will to do all the things I love: play, run, jump, roll around, sing, dance and be happy!

What do you love to do?

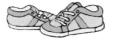

Recommended activities

- Encourage kids to try foods they haven't tasted before. Choose a grain or a pulse (see pages 24-26), for example, mung beans, which most kids love. Find a recipe online, then prepare and eat it together. You can also read about the nutritional value of the food and how it contributes to our bodies. You can try spelt, unprocessed oats, lentils, chickpeas and so on. It is best to teach the kids at an early age to vary foods and to introduce them to other foods than bread, potatoes and pasta. As adults, it will be harder to initiate change, because just like us, they acquire habits. Vegetables, grains and legumes give complete protein and are used by vegetarians to replace meat.

Directions to cook any grains on page 26:
Add a cup of grains to a pot, wash with water and rinse, add a spoon of oil, and cook for a few minutes, add two cups of water, salt, pepper and your choice of herbs, close the lid. When the water is boiling, lower the fire. When the water is absorbed, turn off the fire. You are done! Easy!

Directions to cook any pulses (dried seeds) on page 24-25:
Add a cup of pulses (beans/peas/lentils) to a pot and fill with water to leave overnight. On the day after, drain the water and wash the pulses. Add fresh water to cover the pulses, salt, pepper, and your choice of herbs. Bring to boil then lower the fire. When the pulses are soft and taste edible, drain the water.
Done! Easy!

- Take the kids on a tour of an organic farm and see the food while it is still attached to the ground. Taste it straight from the tree or bush. For example, eating raw, freshly-picked corn or fresh peas is a delicacy. Go on food-related day trips to see how food is grown, and how wine and flour are made.

- Have sliced vegetables and fruits available on the kitchen counter or in the fridge. If anyone of the family gets hungry they have a healthy option.

- Together with the kids, sprout seeds in a pot: green lentils, mung, or any type of legume. **Directions:** Leave some in a closed pot filled with water, overnight. In the morning drain and rinse; cover it with a towel and wait. Locate the pot in a warm area and check once a day for humidity, then stir or add drops of water. In warm areas the sprouts can emerge within a day. Once you see the sprout tail you can remove the towel. It can be kept in a closed container in the fridge for up to two weeks.

The sprouts are delicious, nutritious and very healthy because they are bundles of fine protein, enzymes, vitamins and minerals, and are low in calories. You can add them to salads, mix with rice before serving, add to a sandwich or eat alone as a crispy and tasty snack.

● Grow food like cherry tomatoes, peppers or herbs in a pot or in the garden and enjoy it together.

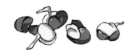

● Take the kids to the market, choose an unfamiliar seasonal vegetable and make a new dish using it. For easy preparation: just stir-fry vegetables with a little water, olive oil, spices and herbs such as dill, parsley, or basil. Always delicious!

● When you're buying packaged food, make sure to notice the list of ingredients.
Know what you are putting into your body.

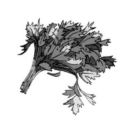

● Just for a day, try to eat only raw fresh food—fruits, nuts, sprouts and vegetables—and find out how it makes you feel.

● Try closing your eyes while you chew, concentrating on the feel and taste of the food. Wait until your mouth is empty before taking another bite.

● Every day, try to eat dark green leaves, like a whole bunch of parsley or baby greens. You can grind them into a spread, adding tomato, avocado, garlic, olive oil and spices then eat it on a slice of bread or with rice or quinoa. People who do this report miraculous changes: healthier children, higher energy and improved vision. Try it for yourself for a week.

● Try to avoid eating wheat for a week and see how it influences your mental clarity, digestion, cravings, sleep and energy level. You can replace the wheat products with rice, potato, corn, rice noodles, bean noodles, rice pasta, polenta, rice crackers. Adding nuts to salads eliminates the need for bread, use pine nuts, pumpkin seeds, sunflower seeds, walnuts, pecans. Add something different every day.

In conclusion

Natural food is food in its natural form. It has had little or no processing. No chemically-engineered materials have been added. For example, vegetables, fruits, rice, oats, lentils, beans, hummus, and probably most dishes your grandmother grew up eating are natural.

Is eating natural food difficult? Not at all! It's just a matter of organization and habits. In fact, the traditional cuisine, and most of the food consumed in the world today is natural. The advanced processed food is a western world thing which brought with it western illnesses.

Nutrition should be simple and intuitive. There are many books and websites on natural diets, with plenty of ideas for diverse meals. Natural nutritionists and naturopathic physicians can help you build you and your family
a balanced daily menu that contains carbohydrates, proteins, fats, vitamins and minerals in the required amounts.

A simple way to start today is to add raw food like a salad
at the beginning of each meal.

Be creative and enjoy.

To your health!

Made in the USA
Columbia, SC
25 July 2021